Get Ripped Ab Muscles

Target Love Handles

Table of Contents

These are some of my other books below, and my website is
www.LosingBellyFatMission.com :

https://www.amazon.com/dp/B06XB4WHZX
http://www.amazon.com/dp/B06X9LXBB8
http://www.amazon.com/dp/B06WLK7497

http://www.amazon.com/dp/B06W54JKQN
http://www.amazon.com/dp/B06X6DJ9K3
http://www.amazon.com/dp/B06WGNJ9N3
http://www.amazon.com/dp/B06W549TBD
http://www.amazon.com/dp/B06VTF5DQJ
http://www.amazon.com/dp/B06WRPSBKK
http://www.amazon.com/dp/B06WD194JR
http://www.amazon.com/dp/B06WCZTK7Y
http://www.amazon.com/dp/B06X3QN1HT
http://www.amazon.com/dp/B01N19WBF2
http://www.amazon.com/dp/B01N2AVECA
http://www.amazon.com/dp/B01N4VZIAV
http://www.amazon.com/dp/B00QJJFS1C
http://www.amazon.com/dp/B01EMNO2MW
http://www.amazon.com/dp/B00SSFWCPA
http://www.amazon.com/dp/1520531230
http://www.amazon.com/dp/B01N4V7SR9
http://www.amazon.com/dp/B00SX58DUI
http://www.amazon.com/dp/B010K7YP62
http://www.amazon.com/dp/B012LAYNNQ
http://www.amazon.com/dp/B00RVX3KY2
http://www.amazon.com/dp/B01MR6SWGW

http://www.amazon.com/dp/B00XF6G4HO
http://www.amazon.com/dp/B01F1472N2
http://www.amazon.com/dp/B00PQ0TUPU
http://www.amazon.com/dp/B00PP8OZJ4
http://www.amazon.com/dp/B00QH7DY4Y
http://www.amazon.com/dp/B01052010G
http://www.amazon.com/dp/B00QDHXN7Q
http://www.amazon.com/dp/B00PO0IQIO

Among others.

Cardio - Lose Weight Through 3 Cardio Exercises

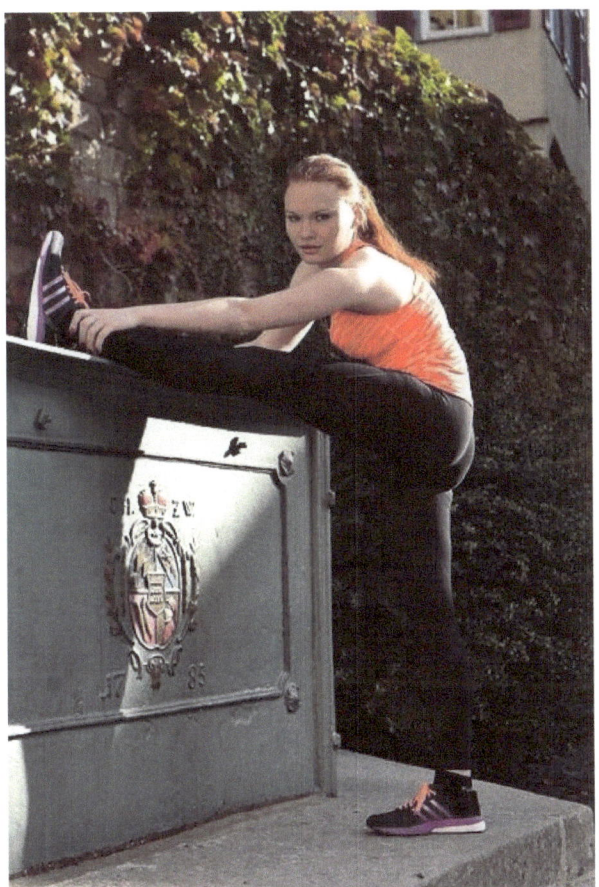

Many body trainers are stating more and more often that it is good to do cardio. There are good reasons for that because it can help you lose weight, have stronger heart and lungs, reduce stress and have many other benefits. You need to know the most common used exercises for a good cardio. They are running, swimming and biking. I am going to talk about each and every one of these activities in this article. The most common cardio exercise is running. For a more efficient result you need to include in your workout uphill running. You will see how hard is to run at a small incline and how fast you will get tired. By doing this type of running you will feel the burning in you muscle leg, your heart rate will increase and you will start to sweat profusely. All this will lead to an increased number of calories that are burned.

Cardio means pushing the limits so it is better if you do a 20 min hard routine instead of a 60 min jogging. The next exercise is even better. One of the best cardio exercises for everyone is swimming. By swimming you will burn more calories than in any other exercise because your entire body is working. Swimming is preferred by elder people because in the water your body has the tendency to lower his tension. A good thing about swimming is that you can choose from different styles. Each one of the swimming styles has his number of calories that are burned if you perform it. If you don't know to swim you can take lessons or do the next cardio exercise.

For most people biking has two purposes. You can move from a place to another and you also do a great cardio exercise. But remember if you just take a nice riding in the park that is not cardio. You need to push your body. A great cardio is to ride your bike uphill. A great thing is that you can do this type of cardio all the year in a gym or at your home because I don't think you are going to ride your bike in the winter when it is snowing. For a good cardio you need to take into consideration each of these exercises.

Running is the best for a nice cardio especial if you do it in the morning. Many people swim just when is hot to cool down but like any other exercise, for a greater result, you need to do it all the time. It is a good thing that you have read this article but for what purpose if you don't include this exercises in your workout?

Losing Weight With Cardio Exercise

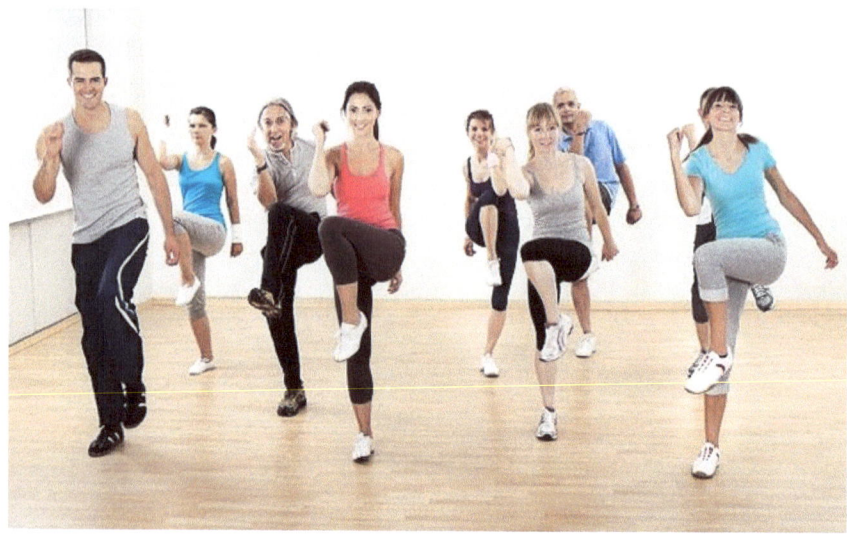

Cardiovascular exercises are quite popular nowadays. The term cardio refers to the heart, which means that this type of exercise involves this vital organ. During cardio exercises, the heart beat is increased and this would result in the body needing greater amount of oxygen. This is the reason why cardio exercise is also called aerobic exercise. Cardiovascular exercises have many benefits for your body. It makes your lungs and heart stronger and free from certain types of diseases. Other benefits include lowering your blood pressure and strengthening and toning your muscles.

One of the best advantages of cardio exercises is that it burns large amounts of calories in your body. This type of exercise is really helpful for those individuals who want to lose weight. Examples of outdoor aerobic exercises include swimming, jogging, biking, running and walking. Indoor aerobic exercise includes using of stair climbers, stationary bicycle, treadmills, elliptical trainers and rowing machines. Cardio exercises are said to be very effective in burning calories in the body. Several weight loss programs have been designed to include different types of cardio exercises. It is though these exercises you would be able to reduce stress, raise the level of energy, strengthen the muscles of the heart, and promote a relaxing sleep. A regular schedule for doing cardio exercises as well as diet modification is an essential aspect in reaching your goal to lose weight.

Proper diet and regular exercises are vital aspects to be physically fit. Exercises will not only help you to lose weight but it will provide many other health benefits. Losing weight is really hard to achieve for some individuals but with proper guidance and motivation, for sure, you will achieve it. Do not dwell on taking diet pills because you can never be sure enough with its side effects. Try to look for weight loss programs which will benefit you the most without suffering any dangerous consequences. Do not force yourself to do heavy exercises such as lifting heavy weights.

Follow a step by step process and try to be patient because surely you will not lose weight with just a wink of an eye. Losing weight is a gradual process that takes time. You will not achieve the desired results if you will try to hasten the process. Stay focused on your goal and be motivated always. You may need someone to encourage you to reach your objective in this regard.

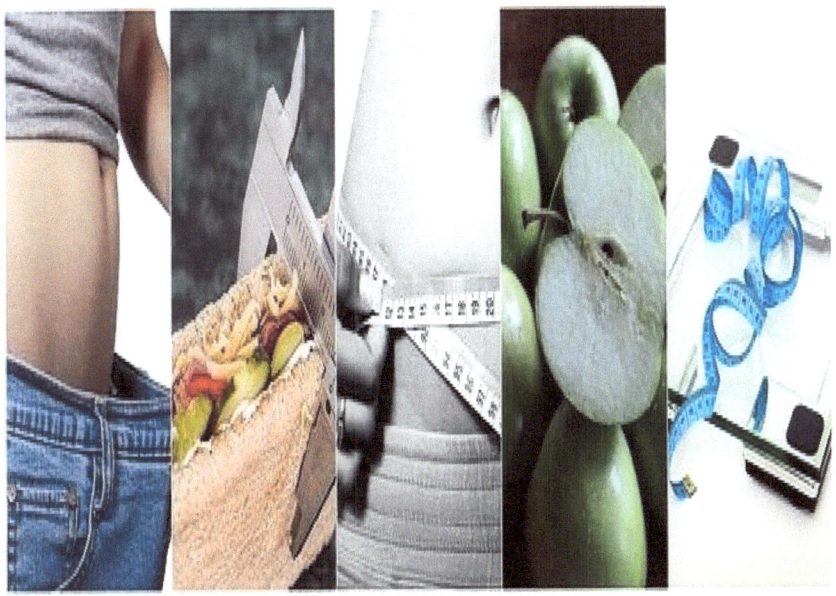

Get up, get moving, get losing - or so spoke your gym teacher in those grueling days of P.E. Looking back through what seems like an endless tunnel of time, you still feel that need to get moving. It's called "gravity," and it's not pretty for most people. If you look out the window, you see the joggers sweating off the weight that you might be putting on, or maybe you're like the author of this article: at a desk for most of the day. (Yikes! Stroke, anyone?) Whatever your reasons for not running, you do understand that you need some exercise.

What are some exercises to do that do not involve running like a track star? Here are some great exercises to try, simply find 15 minutes to dedicate to each one in the beginning until your body gets acclimated to the new habit, be sure to drink plenty of water (8 glasses of water a day won't quite cut the mustard but is a bare minimum to shoot for), and do stretches before and after so you don't leave a nasty email about how you tore your ACL or some hideous thing, and you'll be on your way to looking less like Jabba and more like Luke (this is your brain on Star Wars, my apologies).

Jumping Rope, Riding a Bike To Work or School, Walking, Workout DVDs Like P90X or The Shred Elliptical, Trainers, Jumping Rope. Jumping rope, even for 10 minutes at first, is a clumsy enterprise (speaking, possibly, from experience) - but eventually the hand-eye coordination kicks in. That tends to happen at the same time that the ability to actually complete the full 10 minutes' worth of jumping rope kicks in. At first you may not be able to do but a few jumps before tripping. That's OK, just catch your breath and keep going until your timer goes off.

Helpful Calorie-Blasting Tip: Use a weighted jump rope. They can be found at most any place, and add just a little more kick the workout. The benefit to jumping rope is that your arms as well as your legs and core muscles will get a workout. To kick things in gear, you can use the helpful "cheat sheet" that comes packaged with most weighted ropes, they will show you to try some fancy-pants twists and other steps in order to work your core muscles (that is, your "abs" for you non-gym rats, don't ask when the term was changed - I've yet to hear anyone complain of a "core ache").

Riding a Bike To Work or School

This is a great way to enjoy the outdoors, cause a traffic jam, and get bugs in your eyes. It is also a great way to lose weight, build up endurance, and avoid the pesky jostling about of the high-impact exercises (like running or jumping rope). Calorie-Obliterating Tip: Don't stop. Seriously: you see bikers at stop lights that are in such great shape that it's plainly unfair genetically? They usually try to pedal backwards while staying upright. To lose even more calories, pack 2-3 water bottles with you, for both hydration as well as the added resistance. And to kick it up just a hair more: go mountain biking. Find local hills you can thrash. The changes in elevation and terrain introduce muscle confusion, and gorgeous legs that look decent even in Spandex(R).

Walking

Don't laugh at walking, there are more benefits in walking than in remaining totally sedentary. Walking is great for anyone who has either little equipment, or physical endurance (such as the author of this article at present). Cardio Tip: Walk faster. Find hills to walk up and down, and wear wrist and ankle weights in addition to packing a bottle of water. Try walking 30 minutes at a stretch, at lunch breaks (if you want to stay motivated, take a friend). Workout DVDs Like P90X or The Shred If you haven't seen The Shred or P90X, these are really popular at the moment for good reason: they feature really athletic-looking people who look great on camera. Aside from that, they are also very effective. These are not the only two on the market, but give you the benefit of not needing much equipment other than a few small items (for P90X in particular).

Inexpensive overall, and no need to run: good stuff! Calorie and Fat-Shredding Tips: None - just try them, or products like them - and you'll see they're both sufficient in themselves. Elliptical Trainers Elliptical trainers are a low-impact cardio exercise that will work your entire body (given that you buy a quality elliptical). The benefits are less damage to your joints, and much less likelihood you will become a traffic hazard (can you tell someone has a pet peeve about traffic hazards?).

The advancements in elliptical trainers offer a variety of resistance levels and intensity, as well as providing maximum convenience while you work out. Price ranges from an $88 quasi-elliptical trainer that you can find on Amazon and other places, though it only works your lower body, up to a $7,995.00 Precor AMT100i Experience Series Adaptive Motion Trainer (say that five times fast!). Elliptical provides a great cardio workout while keeping you at home, and are a great way to get and stay in shape without the need to run a single step, which can cause damage to your joints over time.

The Truth About Six Pack Abs - What Many Do Not Know

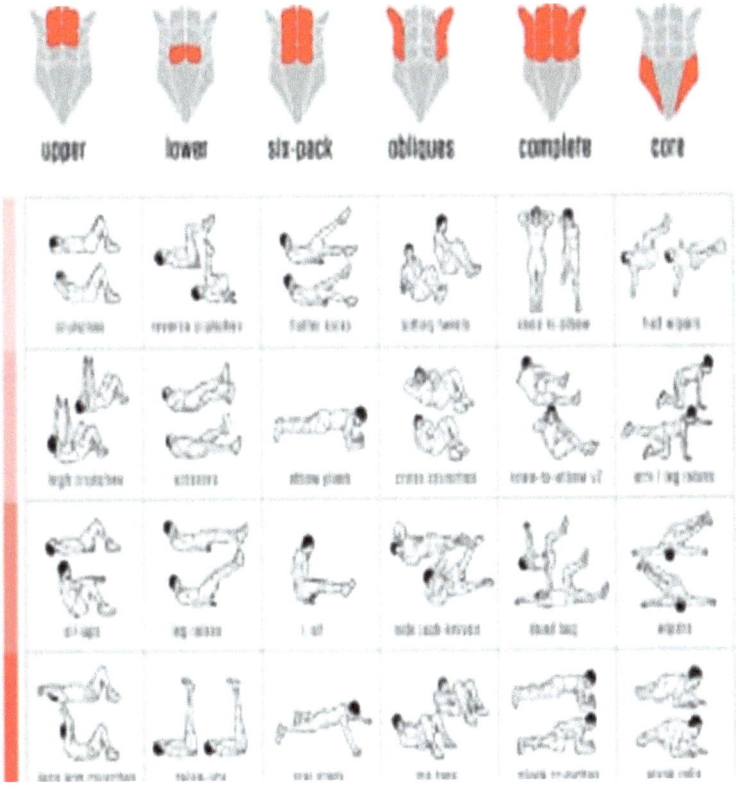

It seems that every human being on the planet is in search for a quick and easy way to get six pack abs fast. The ugly truth is that there is no definitive quick and easy way to get them. Either way you go about it, hard work and dedication is required to reach your ultimate goal, whether it's getting six pack abs or to just lose some weight. Within this article I am going to tell you some common myths about six pack abs, and how you should truly go about getting them.

Common Myths About Six Pack Abs Ab Exercises Is All You Need - This is, for the most part false. Unless you are in shape already with a very low body fat percentage, the truth is everyone has abs. But with most people, their abs are covered with abdominal fat. So along with ab exercises, you need to do cardio exercises to burn fat to show them.

Some People Can Have Six Pack Abs and Some People Can't - I don't know who came up with this myth, but it couldn't be farther from the truth. Like I said above, everyone has abs. The only thing that is stopping them from showing is body fat. Body fat can easily be burned off, but it will take some hard work and dedication. Cardio exercises such as jogging, cycling or even walking can burn off body fat. The key thing here is that you have to stay motivated. There are too many people out there that stick with exercise for a couple of weeks and simply quit.

Losing Weight Through Cardio Exercise

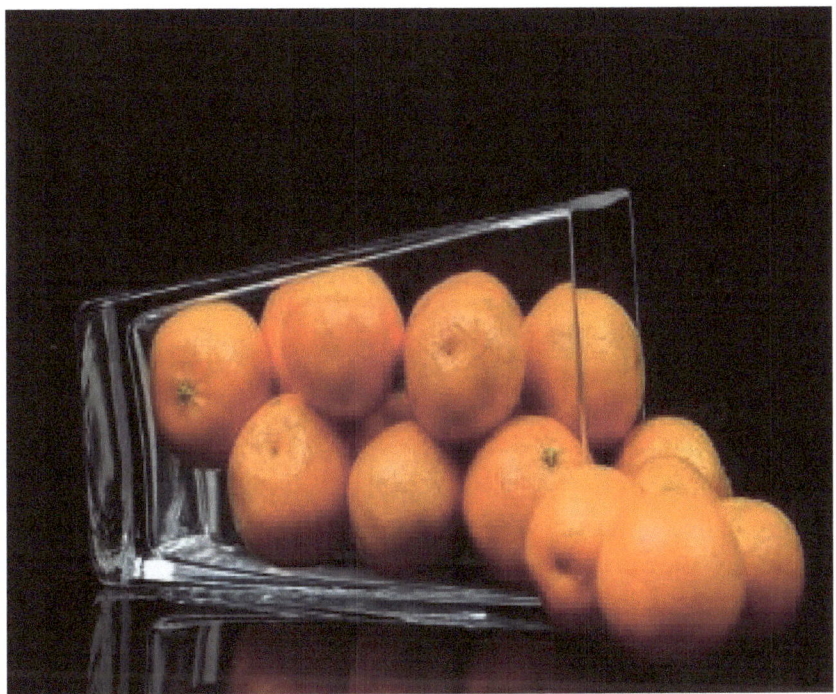

Cardio exercises are one of the best ways in which you can lose weight. They can effectively help to combat weight problems also helps people with maintaining their weight or weight management. Each person has different needs and this should be taken into account when designing a cardio program for each person. Suitable exercises, their intensity and duration should be decided to match a person. Cardio exercises can help a person to lose as much as 100 - 500 calories in one go. As the heart is pumping more oxygen, the calories are burn at a higher rate. In this process, the fat gets burnt easily. A more obese person will torch more calories than a thinner person, given the same duration and intensity of the cardio exercise. They can be done during any time of the week. Along with the cardio exercises, you will also need to follow a specified diet plan that will help you in your aim of losing weight as well.

Cardio exercises aren't meant for everyone. There are high impact and low impact cardio exercises. It's important that you should ask your doctor before proceeding with the exercises. Also if you have recently recovered from heart ailments or any kind of surgery, then you would need the doctor's advice before proceeding with these exercises. The exercises should be done under the strict supervision and guidance of those that are certified trainers. Else you may experience serious injuries while doing the exercises. Since different forms of cardio exercises are meant for different people, there is no single best cardio workout. Walking, jumping, jogging, cycling, swimming, playing outdoor games, cross country skiing are various forms of such exercise. Exercise should be done for at least 5 days in a week for 60 minutes daily to have an impact on weight loss.

Of course other factors such as gender (men lose faster than women), age, genetic makeup, weight and diet make a significant effect on losing weight as well. A normal adult needs as much as 1800 calories a day. If you can spend more calories than the intake, then you can easily lose weight through cardio exercise. You will also need to be regular when doing these exercises. During the phase that you are losing weight, eat home cooked meals as much as possible and substitute low cal foods, salads and fruits in your diet. Have lots of water and refrain from alcohol. Soon you will be able to see your fat melting away.

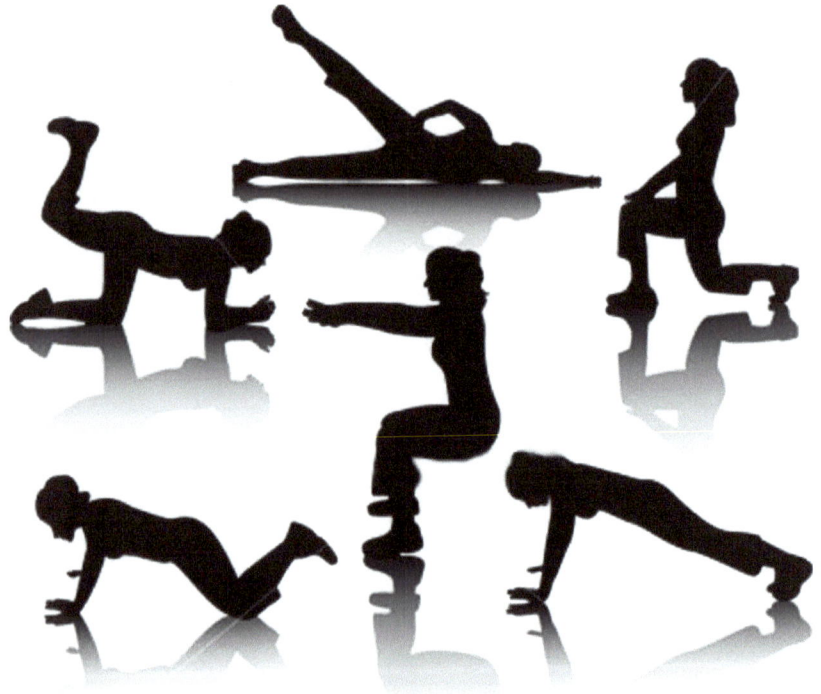

Most of us will reach some point in our lives where we'll be very interested in learning the best exercise to get rid of love handles. It would be a wonderful world if we could all find a way to overcome the inevitable piling on of pounds that come with time, age, and delicious foods to tempt us!:) While it would be great if there were three specific exercises that would immediately melt off your spare tire in a matter of minutes the truth is that there are a few types of exercises that target your love handles and can build leaner muscles that are much better toned when done in combination.

Make Room for Cardio in your Workout Routine The first thing you need to do when creating a workout to target your abdominal area is include regular cardio exercises in your plan. This is actually the best exercise to get rid of love handles you'll find. Why is that? Cardio exercises may not target the specific areas where you want to burn fat but they do a few important things that no other exercises will accomplish.

1) Cardio exercises get the blood pumping. This is important for many reasons. One main reason is that it will move oxygen and nutrients where they need to be while removing toxins and impurities that actually cause the body to retain fat. In other words, when done properly and regularly cardio exercises can actually help you flush the fat from your body. No nasty drinks, detox diets, or painful crunches necessary.

2) Burn baby burn. Seriously, cardio exercises burn calories much more quickly and effectively than other types of exercise. You'll get much more mileage when it comes to calorie burning with a 30 minute cardio exercise three times a week than twice that amount of time doing other exercises that are supposed to target love handles. The more calories you burn through exercise the fewer calories you will find (in the form of unsightly fat) lingering in the side abdominal area.

3) Finally, cardio exercises help you develop stamina. The longer you can sustain the exercise pace or the sooner you can kick your cardio routine up a notch the faster you'll be able to see those firmer abs and long gone love handles in the mirror for yourself. Today is a great day to get started on your journey to better health and a more beautiful body. It just so happens that a great cardio routine is the best exercise to get rid of love handles by far. Start today and see for yourself what it can do to get rid of your love handles.

Benefits of Cardio Exercises

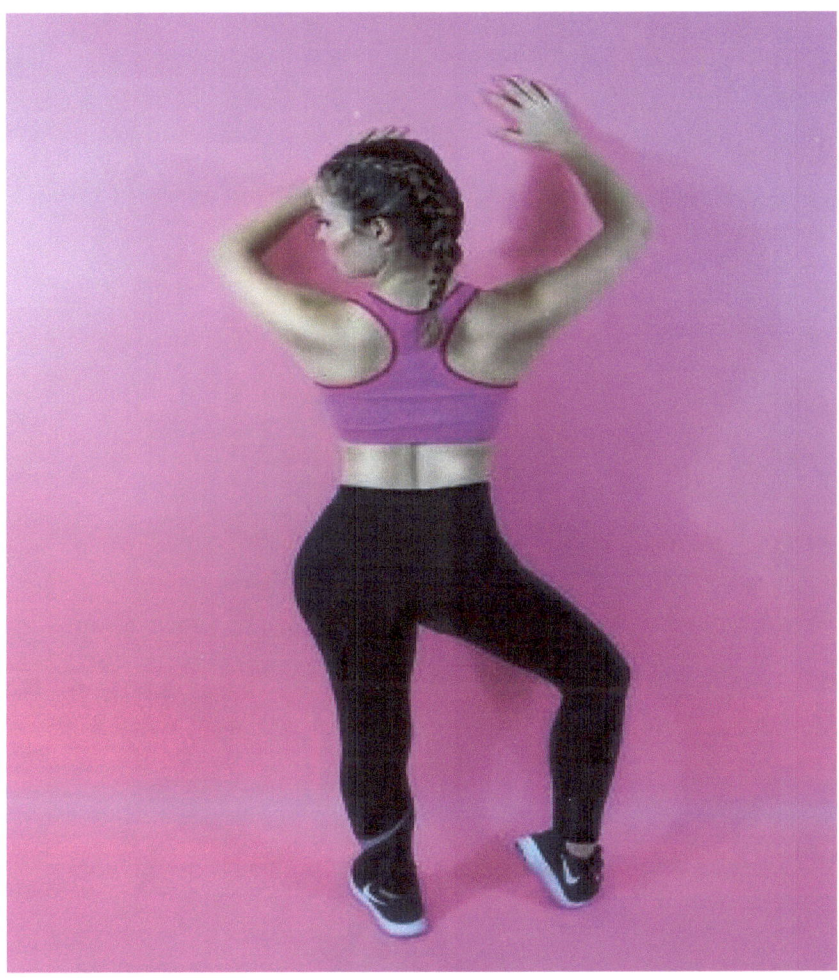

Apart from raising your heart beat and keeping it elated for a while, cardiovascular exercises have some other benefits to your heart muscle and your body in general. It is important to include a cardio workout in your exercise routines as cardio exercises are considered very essential in keeping healthy. The following are some merits of this exercise.

1. It aids greatly in strengthening your heart. This way your heart is able to pump blood easily without getting fatigued.

2. It is also important in strengthening the lungs and by so doing increasing their capacity.

3. It is known to boost the body's metabolism.

4. It is also efficient in burning calories thereby helping one lose weight easily.

5. Studies have shown that cardio exercises are effective in bringing down stress levels of an individual.

6. The exercise also increases body energy giving you more power.

7. By doing a cardio exercise, one can have a good and restful sleep.

Cardio exercise is a very sensitive workout because it involves the heart which is a fragile and a very important organ of the body. It is important to consult a doctor or an exercise consultant before you embark on cardiovascular exercises. However, if you are a beginner it is essential that you start with simple exercises that you can cope with. Cardio exercises for beginners.

As stated above, the first step is to choose an exercise that you enjoy and one that you are comfortable with. One think to consider here is that the best exercise for you is that exercise that you will actually do as opposed to the one you think you should do. Simple exercises such as walking should be a great starting point for you as a beginner. Walking is advisable because you can do it anywhere and anytime. You can also try an exercise that involves continuous movements. Here you can go for swimming, cycling, aerobics, running and others. Continuous movement exercises ensure that your heartbeat is elated for a while.

 After choosing the appropriate activity, it is advisable that you start doing that exercise for about two to three days a week. Ensure to provide a rest day between workouts. During the cardio workout or exercises it is always vital to start with short warm up of about 5-10 minutes. This is then followed by a light cardio which should then be increased gradually to higher heart rate.

After a while it is then important to increase the intensity and pace. Increase the intensity to slightly harder than comfortable. You can use a perceived exertion scale or target heart rate to monitor your intensity with time. Ensure to increase to increase the intensity to a level 5 or 6 on the perceived exertion scale.

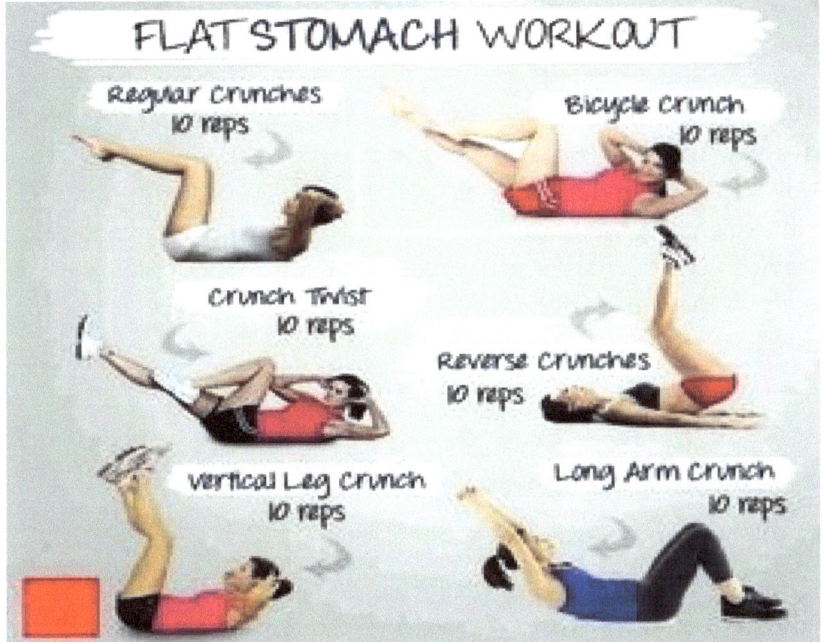

Getting ripped ab muscles is not all that difficult if you know what you are doing. Unfortunately, most people begin working out without having a clue of how to get to where they want to go. The first step on the road to a ripped set of abs begins in the kitchen. Stay away from manufactured and processed foods and stick to lean meats, fish, fruits and veggies and you will be well ahead of the game. The reason most people fail to reach their destination is because they are doing the wrong things to get there.

To lose a pound of fat you must burn 3,500 calories. Most people go about this one of two ways, they do sit ups and other stomach exercises or cardio exercises. Cardio exercises are alright, you'll burn a few hundred calories at a time. Sit ups, crunches and other stomach exercises are fine for building muscle but useless for burning fat and, until you get below 10% body fat for men and 16% for women, you will not see your abs at all. So, it is a matter of burning enough calories to get down to a low enough body fat percentage. The best way to do this is to lift weights. Why? Because muscle weighs more than fat and so the body must work harder and, consequently, burns more fat throughout the day.

A lot of people hear this and start doing curls and working on the weight machines. This is a mistake because the exercises you want to do involve working multiple muscle groups.

Exercises like the clean and jerk, bench press, military press, dumb bell snatches and others are going to cause you to exert such effort that you will actually go into a state of metabolic shock and be a calorie burning furnace for days after the workout.

Abdominal Training!

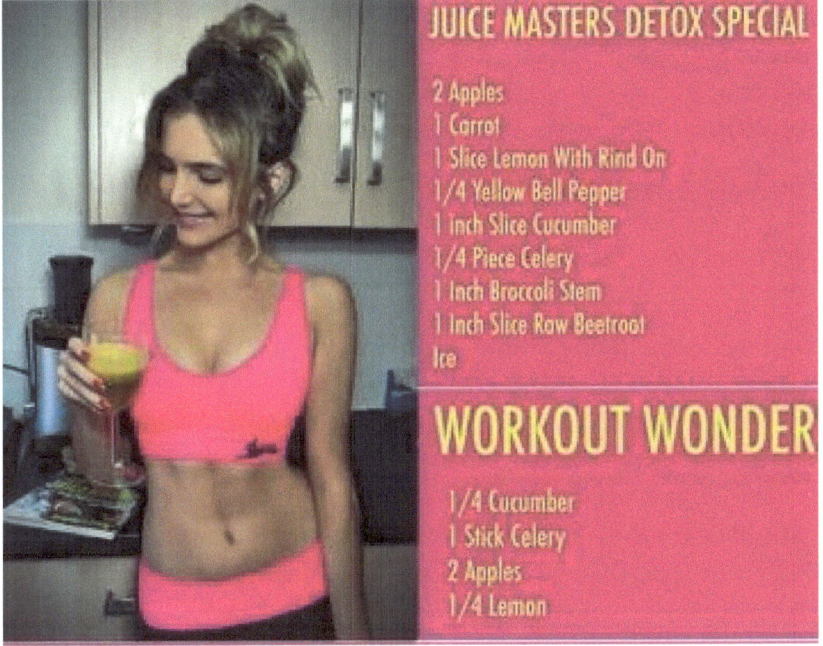

JUICE MASTERS DETOX SPECIAL

2 Apples
1 Carrot
1 Slice Lemon With Rind On
1/4 Yellow Bell Pepper
1 inch Slice Cucumber
1/4 Piece Celery
1 Inch Broccoli Stem
1 Inch Slice Raw Beetroot
Ice

WORKOUT WONDER

1/4 Cucumber
1 Stick Celery
2 Apples
1/4 Lemon

There are an awful lot of misconceptions about abdominal training. Some people can do thousands of sit ups and never see their abs. However, some people do no sit ups at all and have a perfect set of six pack abs. Let me dispel some misconceptions and show you how to get the result you are looking for. When I was 30 pounds overweight, like everyone else I began running and doing stomach crunches. While I burned calories running I just couldn't seem to get rid of the fat around my belly. The misconception that everyone is laboring under is that you can spot reduce belly fat. Not so! To see your abs you must reduce your overall body fat percentage.

While running and other cardio exercises do burn fat and help toward reducing your overall body fat percentage they are not actually the best exercises to do this. Think about it. A pound of fat is 3,500 calories. This is 1,500 calories more than the average person burns in the average day. Even if you spend an hour on the treadmill you will only burn about 500 calories. You've still got 3,000 calories to go to lose a pound of fat. As you can see it is an uphill climb. It was for me until I learned the truth.

The best exercises to do to burn fat are not actually cardio exercises but things like the dead lift, bench press, dips, dumb bell snatches and others. This is because your body exerts so much effort in these that it goes into a state of metabolic shock for days afterward. Your body burns calories at a significantly higher rate. These exercises also work your abs because they stabilize the rest of your body so that you don't need to do ab specific exercises like sit ups and crunches.

These are some of my other books below, and my website is
www.LosingBellyFatMission.com :

https://www.amazon.com/dp/B06XB4WHZX
http://www.amazon.com/dp/B06X9LXBB8
http://www.amazon.com/dp/B06WLK7497
http://www.amazon.com/dp/B06W54JKQN
http://www.amazon.com/dp/B06X6DJ9K3
http://www.amazon.com/dp/B06WGNJ9N3
http://www.amazon.com/dp/B06W549TBD
http://www.amazon.com/dp/B06VTF5DQJ
http://www.amazon.com/dp/B06WRPSBKK
http://www.amazon.com/dp/B06WD194JR
http://www.amazon.com/dp/B06WCZTK7Y
http://www.amazon.com/dp/B06X3QN1HT
http://www.amazon.com/dp/B01N19WBF2
http://www.amazon.com/dp/B01N2AVECA
http://www.amazon.com/dp/B01N4VZIAV
http://www.amazon.com/dp/B00QJJFS1C
http://www.amazon.com/dp/B01EMNO2MW
http://www.amazon.com/dp/B00SSFWCPA
http://www.amazon.com/dp/1520531230
http://www.amazon.com/dp/B01N4V7SR9
http://www.amazon.com/dp/B00SX58DUI
http://www.amazon.com/dp/B010K7YP62
http://www.amazon.com/dp/B012LAYNNQ
http://www.amazon.com/dp/B00RVX3KY2
http://www.amazon.com/dp/B01MR6SWGW
http://www.amazon.com/dp/B00XF6G4HO
http://www.amazon.com/dp/B01F1472N2

http://www.amazon.com/dp/B00PQ0TUPU
http://www.amazon.com/dp/B00PP8OZJ4
http://www.amazon.com/dp/B00QH7DY4Y
http://www.amazon.com/dp/B01052010G
http://www.amazon.com/dp/B00QDHXN7Q
http://www.amazon.com/dp/B00PO0IQIO

Among others.

www.ingramcontent.com/pod-product-compliance
Lightning Source LLC
Chambersburg PA
CBHW050912290526
45792CB00002B/785